© 2019. All rights reserved

No part of this book may electronic, recording, or photocopying without permission of the publisher or author.

Contents

Bipolar 8

Introduction 8

Depression 9

Mania 10

Living with bipolar disorder 11

What causes bipolar disorder? 14

Who's affected? 14

Symptoms 15

Depression 16

Mania 17

Patterns of depression and mania 18

Living with bipolar disorder 20

Symptoms 22

Causes 23

Chemical imbalance in the brain 23

Genetics 25

Triggers.. 25

Diagnosis... 27

Specialist assessment 27

Other tests 29

Treatment 29

Treatment options for bipolar disorder 29

Medication 32

Lithium carbonate 34

Anticonvulsant medicines 37

Valproate... 38

Carbamazepine 40

Lamotrigine 41

Antipsychotic medicines 42

Rapid cycling 44

Learning to recognise triggers 45

Psychological treatment 46

Living with bipolar disorder 51

Staying active and eating well 51

Self-care and self-management 53

Talking about it 56

Services that can help 58

Avoiding drugs and alcohol 60

Money and benefits 61

Dealing with suicidal feelings 65

Self-harm 67

Recommended communities 67

SANE Support Forum 68

What is the Dr. Sebi diet? 69

How to follow the Dr. Sebi diet 71

Potential benefits of the Dr. Sebi diet 73

Foods to avoid 75

Benefits of the Diet 77

Weight Loss 77

Strong Immune System 78

Reduced Risk of Disease 78

Lower Risk of Stroke and Hypertension 79

Tips for Sticking to the Diet 79

Drink Plenty of Water 80

Be Emotionally and Mentally Prepared 81

Don't Give up Snacks 81

Review the Approved Foods 82

Add Whole Foods to Your Diet 82

Cooking is Essential 83

Nutritional Guide and Food List 83

Vegetables 84

Fruits 84

Nuts and Seeds 85

Oils 85

Spices and Seasonings 85

What Not to Eat 85

Dr. Sebi Vegetable List 86

Dr. Sebi Fruit List 88

Dr Sebi Food List Spices and Seasonings 90

Dr Sebi Herbal Teas 92

Dr. Sebi Herb List 93

Why You Need to Cut Back On Processed and Animal-Based Products 94

They are loaded sugar and high fructose corn syrup ..95

They are loaded with refined carbohydrates 96

They are loaded with artificial ingredients.................. 96

They contain components that cause a hyper reward sense in your body 97

Animal Protein Lacks Fiber 98

What You Stand to Gain from Dr Sebi Diet 99

Bipolar

Introduction

Bipolar disorder, formerly known as manic depression, is a condition that affects your moods, which can swing from one extreme to another.

People with bipolar disorder have periods or episodes of:

- depression – feeling very low and lethargic
- mania – feeling very high and overactive (less severe mania is known as hypomania)
- Symptoms of bipolar disorder depend on which mood you're experiencing. Unlike simple mood swings, each extreme episode of bipolar disorder can last for several weeks (or even longer), and

some people may not experience a "normal" mood very often.

Depression

You may initially be diagnosed with clinical depression before having a future manic episode (sometimes years later), after which you may be diagnosed with bipolar disorder.

During an episode of depression, you may have overwhelming feelings of worthlessness, which can potentially lead to thoughts of suicide.

If you're feeling suicidal or having severe depressive symptoms, contact your GP, care co-ordinator or local mental health emergency services as soon as possible.

If you want to talk to someone confidentially, call the Samaritans, free of charge, on 116 123. You can talk to them 24 hours a day, 7 days a week. Alternatively, visit the Samaritans website.

Mania

During a manic phase of bipolar disorder, you may feel very happy and have lots of energy, ambitious plans and ideas. You may spend large amounts of money on things you can't afford and wouldn't normally want.

Not feeling like eating or sleeping, talking quickly and becoming annoyed easily are also common characteristics of this phase.

You may feel very creative and view the manic phase of bipolar as a positive experience. However, you may also experience symptoms of psychosis, where you see or hear things that aren't there or become convinced of things that aren't true.

Living with bipolar disorder

The high and low phases of bipolar disorder are often so extreme that they interfere with everyday life.

However, there are several options for treating bipolar disorder that can make a difference. They aim to control the effects of an episode and help someone with bipolar disorder live life as normally as possible.

The following treatment options are available:

- medication to prevent episodes of mania, hypomania (less severe mania) and depression – these are known as mood stabilisers and are taken every day on a long-term basis
- medication to treat the main symptoms of depression and mania when they occur
- learning to recognise the triggers and signs of an episode of depression or mania
- psychological treatment – such as talking therapy, which can help you deal with depression, and

provides advice about how to improve your relationships
- lifestyle advice – such as doing regular exercise, planning activities you enjoy that give you a sense of achievement, as well as advice on improving your diet and getting more sleep

It's thought using a combination of different treatment methods is the best way to control bipolar disorder.

Help and advice for people with a long-term condition or their carers is also available from charities, support groups and associations.

This includes self-help and self-management advice, and learning to deal with the practical aspects of a long-term condition.

Bipolar disorder and pregnancy

Bipolar disorder, like all other mental health problems, can get worse during pregnancy. However, specialist help is available if you need it.

What causes bipolar disorder?

The exact cause of bipolar disorder is unknown, although it's believed a number of things can trigger an episode. Extreme stress, overwhelming problems and life-changing events are thought to contribute, as well as genetic and chemical factors.

Who's affected?

Bipolar disorder is fairly common and one in every 100 adults will be diagnosed with the condition at some point in their life.

Bipolar disorder can occur at any age, although it often develops between the ages of 15 and 19 and rarely develops after 40. Men and women from all backgrounds are equally likely to develop bipolar disorder.

The pattern of mood swings in bipolar disorder varies widely between people. For example, some people only have a couple of bipolar episodes in their lifetime and are stable in between, while others have many episodes.

Symptoms

Bipolar disorder is characterised by extreme mood swings. These can range from extreme highs (mania) to extreme lows (depression).

Episodes of mania and depression often last for several weeks or months.

Depression

During a period of depression, your symptoms may include:

- feeling sad, hopeless or irritable most of the time
- lacking energy
- difficulty concentrating and remembering things
- loss of interest in everyday activities
- feelings of emptiness or worthlessness
- feelings of guilt and despair
- feeling pessimistic about everything
- self-doubt

- being delusional, having hallucinations and disturbed or illogical thinking
- lack of appetite
- difficulty sleeping
- waking up early
- suicidal thoughts

Mania

The manic phase of bipolar disorder may include:

- feeling very happy, elated or overjoyed
- talking very quickly
- feeling full of energy
- feeling self-important
- feeling full of great new ideas and having important plans
- being easily distracted

- being easily irritated or agitated
- being delusional, having hallucinations and disturbed or illogical thinking
- not feeling like sleeping
- not eating
- doing things that often have disastrous consequences – such as spending large sums of money on expensive and sometimes unaffordable items
- making decisions or saying things that are out of character and that others see as being risky or harmful

Patterns of depression and mania

If you have bipolar disorder, you may have episodes of depression more regularly than episodes of mania, or vice versa.

Between episodes of depression and mania, you may sometimes have periods where you have a "normal" mood.

The patterns aren't always the same and some people may experience:

rapid cycling – where a person with bipolar disorder repeatedly swings from a high to low phase quickly without having a "normal" period in between

mixed state – where a person with bipolar disorder experiences symptoms of depression and mania together; for example, overactivity with a depressed mood

If your mood swings last a long time but aren't severe enough to be classed as bipolar disorder, you may be diagnosed with cyclothymia (a mild form of bipolar disorder).

Living with bipolar disorder

Bipolar disorder is a condition of extremes. A person with the condition may be unaware they're in the manic phase.

After the episode is over, they may be shocked at their behaviour. However, at the time, they may believe other people are being negative or unhelpful.

Some people with bipolar disorder have more frequent and severe episodes than others. The extreme nature of the condition means staying in a job may be difficult and relationships may become strained. There's also an increased risk of suicide.

During episodes of mania and depression, someone with bipolar disorder may experience strange sensations, such as seeing, hearing or smelling things that aren't there (hallucinations).

They may also believe things that seem irrational to other people (delusions). These types of symptoms are known as psychosis or a psychotic episode.

Symptoms

Bipolar disorder is characterised by extreme mood swings. These can range from extreme highs (mania) to extreme lows (depression).

If your mood swings last a long time but aren't severe enough to be classed as bipolar disorder, you may be diagnosed with cyclothymia (a mild form of bipolar disorder).

During episodes of mania and depression, someone with bipolar disorder may experience strange sensations, such as seeing, hearing or smelling things that aren't there (hallucinations).

They may also believe things that seem irrational to other people (delusions). These types of symptoms are known as psychosis or a psychotic episode.

Causes

The exact cause of bipolar disorder is unknown. Experts believe there are a number of factors that work together to make a person more likely to develop the condition.

These are thought to be a complex mix of physical, environmental and social factors.

Chemical imbalance in the brain

Bipolar disorder is widely believed to be the result of chemical imbalances in the brain.

The chemicals responsible for controlling the brain's functions are called neurotransmitters and include noradrenaline, serotonin and dopamine.

There's some evidence that if there's an imbalance in the levels of one or more neurotransmitters, a person may develop some symptoms of bipolar disorder.

For example, there's evidence that episodes of mania may occur when levels of noradrenaline are too high, and episodes of depression may be the result of noradrenaline levels becoming too low.

Genetics

It's also thought bipolar disorder is linked to genetics, as the condition seems to run in families. The family members of a person with the condition have an increased risk of developing it themselves.

However, no single gene is responsible for bipolar disorder. Instead, a number of genetic and environmental factors are thought to act as triggers.

Triggers

A stressful circumstance or situation often triggers the symptoms of bipolar disorder. Examples of stressful triggers include:

- the breakdown of a relationship
- physical, sexual or emotional abuse
- the death of a close family member or loved one

These types of life-altering events can cause episodes of depression at any time in a person's life.

Bipolar disorder may also be triggered by:

- physical illness
- sleep disturbances
- overwhelming problems in everyday life – such as problems with money, work or relationships

Diagnosis

If your GP thinks you may have bipolar disorder, they'll usually refer you to a psychiatrist (a medically qualified mental health specialist).

If your illness puts you at risk of harming yourself, your GP will arrange an appointment immediately.

Specialist assessment

You'll be assessed by the psychiatrist at your appointment. They'll ask you a few questions to determine if you have bipolar disorder. If you do, they'll decide what treatments are most suitable.

During the assessment, you'll be asked about your symptoms and when you first experienced them. The psychiatrist will also ask about how you feel leading up to and during an episode of mania or depression, and if you have thoughts about harming yourself.

The psychiatrist will also want to know about your medical background and family history, especially whether any of your relatives have had bipolar disorder.

If someone else in your family has the condition, the psychiatrist may want to talk to them. However, they'll ask for your agreement before doing so.

Other tests

Depending on your symptoms, you may also need tests to see whether you have a physical problem, such as an underactive thyroid or an overactive thyroid.

If you have bipolar disorder, you'll need to visit your GP regularly for a physical health check.

Treatment

Treatment for bipolar disorder aims to reduce the severity and number of episodes of depression and mania to allow as normal a life as possible.

Treatment options for bipolar disorder

If a person isn't treated, episodes of bipolar-related mania can last for between three and six months.

Episodes of depression tend to last longer, for between six and 12 months.

However, with effective treatment, episodes usually improve within about three months.

Most people with bipolar disorder can be treated using a combination of different treatments. These can include one or more of the following:

medication to prevent episodes of mania, hypomania (less severe mania) and depression – these are known as mood stabilisers and are taken every day on a long-term basis

medication to treat the main symptoms of depression and mania when they occur

learning to recognise the triggers and signs of an episode of depression or mania

psychological treatment – such as talking therapies, which help you deal with depression and provide advice on how to improve relationships

lifestyle advice – such as doing regular exercise, planning activities you enjoy that give you a sense of achievement, and advice on improving your diet and getting more sleep

Read more about living with bipolar disorder

Most people with bipolar disorder can receive most of their treatment without having to stay in hospital.

However, hospital treatment may be needed if your symptoms are severe, or if you're being treated under the Mental Health Act, as there's a danger you may self-harm or hurt others.

In some circumstances, you could have treatment in a day hospital and return home at night.

Medication

Several medications are available to help stabilise mood swings. These are commonly referred to as mood stabilisers and include:

lithium carbonate

anticonvulsant medicines

antipsychotic medicines

If you're already taking medication for bipolar disorder and you develop depression, your GP will check you're taking the correct dose. If you aren't, they'll change it.

Episodes of depression are treated slightly differently in bipolar disorder, as the use of antidepressants alone may lead to a hypomanic relapse.

Most guidelines suggest depression in bipolar disorder can be treated with just a mood stabiliser. However, antidepressants are commonly used alongside a mood stabiliser or antipsychotic.

If your GP or psychiatrist recommends you stop taking medication for bipolar disorder, the dose should be gradually reduced over at least four weeks, and up to three months if you are taking an antipsychotic or lithium.

If you have to stop taking lithium for any reason, see your GP about taking an antipsychotic or valproate instead.

Lithium carbonate

In the UK, lithium carbonate (often referred to as just lithium) is the medication most commonly used to treat bipolar disorder.

Lithium is a long-term method of treatment for episodes of mania, hypomania and depression. It's usually prescribed for at least six months.

If you're prescribed lithium, stick to the prescribed dose and don't stop taking it suddenly (unless told to by your doctor).

For lithium to be effective, the dosage must be correct. If it's incorrect, you may get side effects such as diarrhoea and vomiting. However, tell your doctor immediately if you have side effects while taking lithium.

You'll need regular blood tests at least every three months while taking lithium. This is to make sure your lithium levels aren't too high or too low.

Your kidney and thyroid function will also need to be checked every two to three months if the dose of lithium is being adjusted, and every 12 months in all other cases.

While you're taking lithium, avoid using non-steroidal anti-inflammatory drugs (NSAIDs), such as ibuprofen, unless they're prescribed by your GP.

In the UK, lithium and the antipsychotic medicine aripiprazole are currently the only medications licensed for use in adolescents with bipolar disorder who are aged 13 or over.

However, the Royal College of Paediatrics and Child Health states that unlicensed medicines may be prescribed for children if there are no suitable alternatives and their use can be justified by expert agreement.

Anticonvulsant medicines

Anticonvulsant medicines include:

- valproate
- carbamazepine
- lamotrigine

These medicines are sometimes used to treat episodes of mania. They're also long-term mood stabilisers.

Anticonvulsant medicines are often used to treat epilepsy, but they're also effective in treating bipolar disorder.

A single anticonvulsant medicine may be used, or they may be used in combination with lithium when the condition doesn't respond to lithium on its own.

Valproate

Valproate isn't usually prescribed for women of childbearing age because there's a risk of physical defects to babies such as spina bifida, heart abnormalities and cleft lip. There may also be an increased risk of developmental problems such as lower intellectual abilities, poor speaking and understanding, memory problems, autistic spectrum disorders and delayed walking and talking.

Learn more about the risks of valproate medicines during pregnancy

In women, your GP may decide to use valporate if there's no alternative or if you've been assessed and it's unlikely you'll respond to other treatments, although they'll need to check you're using a reliable contraception and advise you on the risks of taking the medicine during pregnancy.

If you're prescribed valproate, you'll need to visit your GP to have a blood count when you begin the medication, and then again six months later.

Carbamazepine

Carbamazepine is usually only prescribed on the advice of an expert in bipolar disorder. To begin with, the dose will be low and then gradually increased.

Your progress will be carefully monitored if you're taking other medication, including the contraceptive pill.

Blood tests to check your liver and kidney function will be carried out when you start taking carbamazepine, and again after six months.

You'll also need to have a blood count at the start and after six months, and you may also have your weight and height monitored.

Lamotrigine

If you're prescribed lamotrigine, you'll usually be started on a low dose, which will be increased gradually.

See your GP immediately if you're taking lamotrigine and develop a rash. You'll need to have an annual health check, but other tests aren't usually needed.

Women who are taking the contraceptive pill should talk to their GP about taking a different method of contraception.

Antipsychotic medicines

Antipsychotic medicines are sometimes prescribed to treat episodes of mania or hypomania. Antipsychotic medicines include:

- aripiprazole
- olanzapine
- quetiapine
- risperidone

They may also be used as a long-term mood stabiliser. Quetiapine may also be used for long-term bipolar depression.

Antipsychotic medicines can be particularly useful if symptoms are severe or behaviour is disturbed. As antipsychotics can cause side effects – such as blurred vision, dry mouth, constipation and weight gain – the initial dose will usually be low.

If you're prescribed an antipsychotic medicine, you'll need to have regular health checks at least every three months, but possibly more often, particularly if you have diabetes. If your symptoms don't improve, you may be offered lithium and valproate as well.

Aripiprazole is also recommended by the National Institute for Health and Care Excellence (NICE) as an option for treating moderate to severe manic episodes in adolescents with bipolar disorder.

Rapid cycling

You may be prescribed a combination of lithium and valproate if you experience rapid cycling (where you quickly change from highs to lows without a "normal" period in between).

If this doesn't help, you may be offered lithium on its own or a combination of lithium, valproate and lamotrigine.

However, you won't usually be prescribed an antidepressant unless an expert in bipolar disorder has recommended it.

Learning to recognise triggers

If you have bipolar disorder, you can learn to recognise the warning signs of an approaching episode of mania or depression.

A community mental health worker, such as a psychiatric nurse, may be able to help you identify your early signs of relapse from your history.

This won't prevent the episode occurring, but it will allow you to get help in time.

This may mean making some changes to your treatment, perhaps by adding an antidepressant or antipsychotic medicine to the mood-stabilising medication you're already taking. Your GP or specialist can advise you on this.

Psychological treatment

Some people find psychological treatment helpful when used alongside medication in between episodes of mania or depression. This may include:

psychoeducation – to find out more about bipolar disorder

cognitive behavioural therapy (CBT) – this is most useful when treating depression

family therapy – a type of psychotherapy that focuses on family relationships (such as marriage) and encourages everyone within the family or relationship to work together to improve mental health

Psychological treatment usually consists of around 16 sessions. Each session lasts an hour and takes place over a period of six to nine months.

Pregnancy

The management of bipolar disorder in women who are pregnant, or those who are trying to conceive, is complex and challenging.

One of the main problems is the risks of taking medication during pregnancy aren't always that well understood.

The National Institute for Health and Care Excellence (NICE) recommends that the risks of treating or not treating women with bipolar disorder during pregnancy should be fully discussed.

NICE also recommends that specialist mental health services work closely with maternity services.

A written plan for managing the treatment of a pregnant woman with bipolar disorder should be developed as soon as possible.

The plan should be drawn up with the patient, her partner, her obstetrician (pregnancy specialist), midwife, GP and health visitor.

The following medication isn't routinely prescribed for pregnant women with bipolar disorder:

valproate – there's a risk to the foetus and the subsequent development of the child

carbamazepine – it has limited effectiveness and there's risk of harm to the foetus

lithium – there's a risk of harm to the foetus, such as cardiac problems

lamotrigine – there's a risk of harm to the foetus

paroxetine – there's a risk of harm to the foetus, such as cardiovascular malformations

benzodiazepines – if used long term, there are risks during the pregnancy and immediately after the birth, such as cleft palate and floppy baby syndrome

If you become pregnant while taking medication prescribed to treat bipolar disorder, it's important that you don't stop taking it until you've discussed it with your doctor.

If medication is prescribed for bipolar disorder after the baby is born, it may also affect a mother's decision to breastfeed her child. Your pharmacist, midwife or mental health team can give you advice based on your circumstances.

Living with bipolar disorder

Although it's usually a long-term condition, effective treatments for bipolar disorder, combined with self-help techniques, can limit the condition's impact on your everyday life.

Staying active and eating well

Eating well and keeping fit are important for everyone. Exercise can also help reduce the symptoms of bipolar disorder, particularly depressive symptoms.

It may also give you something to focus on and provide a routine, which is important for many people.

A healthy diet, combined with exercise, may also help limit weight gain, which is a common side effect of medical treatments for bipolar disorder.

Some treatments also increase the risk of developing diabetes, or worsen the illness in people that already have it. Maintaining a healthy weight and exercising are an important way of limiting that risk.

You should have a check-up at least once a year to monitor your risk of developing cardiovascular disease or diabetes.

This will include recording your weight, checking your blood pressure and having any appropriate blood tests.

Read more information about losing weight and improving fitness

Self-care and self-management

Self-care

Self-care is an essential part of daily life. It involves taking responsibility for your own health and wellbeing with support from the people involved in your care.

It includes:

- staying fit and maintaining good physical and mental health
- preventing illness or accidents

- caring more effectively for minor ailments and long-term conditions

People with long-term conditions can benefit enormously from being helped with self-care. They can live longer, have less pain, anxiety, depression and fatigue, have a better quality of life, and be more active and independent.

Self-management programmes

Self-management programmes aim to help people with bipolar disorder take an active part in their own recovery so they're not controlled by their condition.

One course run by Bipolar UK aims to teach people with bipolar disorder how to manage their illness. The programme includes information about:

- triggers and warning signs
- coping strategies and self-medication
- support networks and action plans
- maintaining a healthy lifestyle
- drawing up an advance decision
- complementary therapies
- action plans

There are other courses, such as those run by Self Management UK, for mild to moderate mental health conditions.

Courses such as these help people who may feel distressed and uncertain about their bipolar disorder improve their own lives.

Talking about it

Some people with bipolar disorder find it easy to talk to family and friends about their condition and its effects. Other people find it easier to turn to charities and support groups.

Many organisations run self-help groups that can put you in touch with other people with the condition. This enables people to share helpful ideas and helps them realise they're not alone in feeling the way they do. These organisations also provide online support in forums and blogs.

Some useful charities, support groups and associations include:

- Bipolar UK
- Carers UK
- Mind
- Rethink
- Samaritans
- SANE

Talking therapies are useful for managing bipolar disorder, particularly during periods of stability.

Services that can help

You may be involved with many different services during treatment for bipolar disorder. Some are accessed through referral from your GP, others through your local authority.

These services may include:

Community mental health teams (CMHT) – these provide the main part of local specialist mental health services. They offer assessment, treatment and social care to people with bipolar disorder and other mental illnesses.

Early intervention teams – these provide early identification and treatment for people who have the first symptoms of psychosis. Your GP may be able to refer you directly to an early intervention team.

Crisis services – these allow people to be treated at home, instead of in hospital, for an acute episode. These are specialist mental health teams that deal with crises that occur outside normal office hours.

Acute day hospital – these are an alternative to inpatient care in a hospital. You can visit every day or as often as you need.

Assertive outreach teams – these deliver intensive treatment and rehabilitation in the community for people with severe mental health problems, providing rapid help in a crisis. Staff often visit people at home and liaise with other services, such as your GP or social services. They can also help with practical problems, such as helping to find housing and work, or doing your shopping and cooking.

Avoiding drugs and alcohol

Some people with bipolar disorder use alcohol or illegal drugs to try to take away their pain and distress. Both have well-known harmful physical and social effects and are not a substitute for effective treatment and good healthcare.

Some people with bipolar disorder find they can stop misusing alcohol and drugs once they're using effective treatment.

Others may have separate but related problems of alcohol and drug abuse, which may need to be treated separately.

Avoiding alcohol and illegal drugs is an important part of recovery from episodes of manic, hypomanic or depressive symptoms, and can help you gain stability.

Money and benefits

It's important to avoid too much stress, including work-related stress. If you're employed, you may be able to work shorter hours or in a more flexible way, particularly if job pressure triggers your symptoms.

Under the Disability Discrimination Act 1995, all employers must make reasonable adjustments to make the employment of people with disabilities possible. This can include people with a diagnosis of bipolar disorder or other mental illnesses.

A range of benefits is available to people with bipolar disorder who can't work as a result of their mental illness. These may include:

- Attendance Allowance
- Carer's Allowance
- Council Tax Benefit
- Disability Living Allowance
- Housing Benefit
- Incapacity Benefit
- Statutory Sick Pay

Care Information Scotland: Money

Living with or caring for someone with bipolar disorder

People living with or caring for someone with bipolar disorder can have a tough time. During episodes of illness, the personalities of people with bipolar disorder may change, and they may become abusive or even violent.

Sometimes social workers and the police may become involved. Relationships and family life are likely to feel the strain.

If you're the Named Person (as defined by the Mental Health (Scotland) Act 2015) of a person with bipolar disorder, you have certain rights that can be used to protect the person's interests.

These include requesting that the local social services authority asks an approved mental health professional to consider whether the person with bipolar disorder should be detained in hospital (also known as "sectioning").

You may feel at a loss if you're caring for someone with bipolar disorder. Finding a support group and talking to other people in a similar situation might help.

If you're having relationship or marriage difficulties, you can contact specialist relationship counsellors, who can talk things through with you and your partner.

Dealing with suicidal feelings

Having suicidal thoughts is a common depressive symptom of bipolar disorder. Without treatment, these thoughts may get stronger.

Some research has shown the risk of suicide for people with bipolar disorder is 15 to 20 times greater than the general population.

Studies have also shown that as many as 25-50% of people with bipolar disorder attempt suicide at least once.

The risk of suicide seems to be higher earlier in the illness, so early recognition and help may prevent it.

If you're feeling suicidal or you're having severe depressive symptoms, contact your GP, care co-ordinator or the local mental health emergency services as soon as possible.

If you can't or don't want to contact these people, contact the Samaritans on 116 123. You can call them 24 hours a day, seven days a week.

Alternatively, visit the Samaritans website or email jo@samaritans.org.

Self-harm

Self-harm (sometimes called self-injury) is often a symptom of mental health problems such as bipolar disorder.

For some people, self-harm is a way of gaining control over their lives or temporarily distracting themselves from mental distress. It may not be related to suicide or attempted suicide.

Recommended communities

Online communities help you talk to people, share your experiences and learn from others.

The SANE Support Forum allows people to share their feelings and provide mutual support to anyone with mental health issues, as well as their friends and family.

SANE Support Forum

Bipolar UK, a national charity, also runs an online discussion forum for people with bipolar disorder, their families and carers.

What is the Dr. Sebi diet?

This diet is based on the African Bio-Mineral Balance theory and was developed by the self-educated herbalist Alfredo Darrington Bowman — better known as Dr. Sebi. Despite his name, Dr. Sebi was not a medical doctor and did not hold a PhD.

He designed this diet for anyone who wishes to naturally cure or prevent disease and improve their overall health without relying on conventional Western medicine.

According to Dr. Sebi, disease is a result of mucus build-up in an area of your body. For example, a build-up of mucus in the lungs is pneumonia, while excess mucus in the pancreas is diabetes.

He argues that diseases cannot exist in an alkaline environment and begin to occur when your body becomes too acidic.

By strictly following his diet and using his proprietary costly supplements, he promises to restore your body's natural alkaline state and detoxify your diseased body.

The diet consists of a specific list of approved vegetables, fruits, grains, nuts, seeds, oils, and herbs. As animal products are not permitted, the Dr. Sebi diet is considered a vegan diet.

Sebi claimed that for your body to heal itself, you must follow the diet consistently for the rest of your life.

How to follow the Dr. Sebi diet

The rules of the Dr. Sebi diet are very strict and outlined on his website.

According to Dr. Sebi's nutritional guide, you must follow these key rules:

Rule 1. You must only eat foods listed in the nutritional guide.

Rule 2. Drink 1 gallon (3.8 liters) of water every day.

Rule 3. Take Dr. Sebi's supplements an hour before medications.

Rule 4. No animal products are permitted.

Rule 5. No alcohol is allowed.

Rule 6. Avoid wheat products and only consume the "natural-growing grains" listed in the guide.

Rule 7. Avoid using a microwave to prevent killing your food.

Rule 8. Avoid canned or seedless fruits.

There are no specific nutrient guidelines. However, this diet is low in protein, as it prohibits beans, lentils, and animal and soy products. Protein is an important nutrient needed for strong muscles, skin, and joints.

Additionally, you're expected to purchase Dr. Sebi's cell food products, which are supplements that promise to cleanse your body and nourish your cells.

It's recommended to buy the "all-inclusive" package, which contains 20 different products that are claimed to cleanse and restore your entire body at the fastest rate possible.

Besides this, no specific supplement recommendations are provided. Instead, you're expected to order any supplement that matches your health concerns.

Potential benefits of the Dr. Sebi diet

One benefit of the Dr. Sebi diet is its strong emphasis on plant-based foods.

The diet promotes eating a large number of vegetables and fruit, which are high in fiber, vitamins, minerals, and plant compounds.

Diets rich in vegetables and fruit have been associated with reduced inflammation and oxidative stress, as well as protection against many diseases.

In a study in 65,226 people, those who ate 7 or more servings of vegetables and fruit per day had a 25% and 31% lower incidence of cancer and heart disease, respectively.

Furthermore, most people are not eating enough produce. In a 2017 report, 9.3% and 12.2% of people met the recommendations for vegetables and fruit, respectively.

Moreover, the Dr. Sebi diet promotes eating fiber-rich whole grains and healthy fats, such as nuts, seeds, and plant oils. These foods have been linked to a lower risk of heart disease.

Finally, diets that limit ultra-processed foods are associated with better overall diet quality

Foods to avoid

Any foods that are not included in the Dr. Sebi nutrition guide are not permitted, such as:

- canned fruit or vegetables

- seedless fruit
- eggs
- dairy
- fish
- red meat
- poultry
- soy products
- processed food, including take-out or restaurant food
- fortified foods
- wheat
- sugar (besides date sugar and agave syrup)
- alcohol
- yeast or foods risen with yeast
- foods made with baking powder

Furthermore, many vegetables, fruits, grains, nuts, and seeds are banned on the diet.

Only foods listed in the guide may be eaten.

Benefits of the Diet

Minimizing acid in foods helps to decrease mucus in the body, which creates an alkaline environment within your body that makes it very difficult for disease to form.

Weight Loss

This part is self-explanatory. Weight loss is bound to happen when following the diet because this diet consists of natural vegetables, fruits, grains, nuts, and legumes.

It eliminates waste, dairy, meat, and processed food, so naturally, your body will lose weight. This diet serves as a cleanse and reaps many benefits. Your body will thank you!

Strong Immune System

A weak immune system is the result of illnesses and diseases. Some claim that they have strengthened their immune system and have been healed of certain ailments by following this diet consistently.

Reduced Risk of Disease

Acidic foods erode the mucous membrane of the cells and inner walls of the body which leads to a compromised system that makes disease possible. As a result, eating alkaline foods can reduce the risk of disease and help your body in getting what it needs to feed the good cells.

Lower Risk of Stroke and Hypertension

According to the National Institute of Health (NIH), first line therapies for all stages of hypertension include exercise and weight loss. However, results from one small cross-sectional study suggest that a plant-based diet is the more important intervention.

Everyday Health has also discussed the benefits of a plant based diet, stating that a plant-based diet can decrease plaque in the blood vessels and lower risk of diabetes and stroke

Tips for Sticking to the Diet

Like any other diet you try, this one will take time and effort! While it may be difficult at first, your body will slowly get used to this new way of eating. You will begin to feel more energized as you eliminate all the bad foods you may have consumed in the past. Down below are a few suggestions and guidelines to follow to make this the most enjoyable experience possible.

Drink Plenty of Water

According to Bowman, people should be drinking at least a gallon of water per day. This is essential to making this alkaline diet work to the best of its ability. Alfredo recommends natural spring water as opposed to water softeners or water from a reverse osmosis system. Other health organizations and nutritional experts suggest a gallon of water per day too. Keep in mind that water removes waste from the body while assisting in the absorption of nutrients and cushioning joints and organs.

Be Emotionally and Mentally Prepared

It is extremely likely that you have formed some strong habits eating certain types of foods daily that may make it very hard to break or change your diet. Your family and friends may also become a hindrance when trying to carry out this diet. Before beginning this plan, spend some time thinking about why you want to change your eating and the obstacles, both mental and emotional, that you will face.

Don't Give up Snacks

Yes, you heard right! While you do not have to give up snacks, you do have to snack the right way. This means instead of reaching for a bag of potato chips, eat a piece of fruit or create snacks based on the recommended nutritional guide.

Review the Approved Foods

Do your best not to stray from the list of approved foods as it can hinder your results. While it may seem too difficult at first to eat from the selected list, you'll soon find it's easier than thought especially if you are prepared mentally.

Add Whole Foods to Your Diet

Do your best to substitute packaged foods with whole foods in your diet on a regular basis. You want to avoid packaged foods because they are full of additives, which can be very addictive especially since many have refined sugar that causes food cravings.

Cooking is Essential

You will quickly find that it's necessary to cook when trying this diet. The guides guides offer alkaline food recipes to make this process easier. His guides walk you step by step through each alkaline meal. After you begin preparing your own meals, you'll see how you can take your favorite dishes and prepare them using approved ingredients.

Nutritional Guide and Food List

You may be wondering what foods you can eat. While it seems like your options are limited, they are not and the diet is simple and achievable.

Most of the non-hybrid foods on the nutritional guide are listed below.

Vegetables

Amaranth Greens, Wild Arugula, Asparagus, Bell Peppers, Mexican Squash or Chayote, Garbanzo Beans (chickpeas), Kale, Lettuce (except for Iceberg), Mushrooms, Mexican Cactus or Nopales, Okra, Onions, Squash, Tomato (cherry and plum), Zucchini

Fruits

Apples, Bananas, Orange, Berries, Cantaloupe, Cherries, Figs, Grapes -seeded, Limes, Mango, Melons -seeded, Papayas, Plums, Peaches, Pears, Prickly Pear (Cactus Fruit), Prunes, Raisins -seeded, Tamarind

Nuts and Seeds

Brazil Nuts, Hemp Seed, Raw Sesame Seeds, Walnuts

Oils

Olive Oil, Coconut Oil, Grapeseed Oil, Hempseed Oil, Avocado Oil

Spices and Seasonings

Basil, Cayenne, Cloves, Dill, Habanero, Onion Powder, Oregano, Pure Sea Salt, Sage, Thyme

What Not to Eat

Meat, dairy (eggs, milk, etc), garlic, white sugar, man-made food

Because this diet is strict, you may find the first few days to be extremely challenging.

Lucky for you we have a page with recipes and there are also tons of videos on Youtube.

Popular recipes include meatless meatballs, alkaline based noodle recipe, and fluffy gluten-free waffles.

Dr. Sebi Vegetable List

As with all his electric foods, Dr. Sebi held the belief that people should eat non-GMO foods. This includes fruits and vegetables that have been made seedless, or altered to contain more vitamins and minerals than they do naturally. The Dr. Sebi list of vegetables is rather large and diverse, with plenty of options to create different dynamic meals. This list includes:

- Amaranth

- Arame
- Avocado
- Bell Pepper
- Chayote
- Cherry and Plum Tomato
- Cucumber
- Dandelion Greens
- Dulse
- Garbanzo Beans
- Hijiki
- Izote flower and leaf
- Kale
- Lettuce except iceberg
- Mushrooms except Shitake
- Nopales
- Nori

- Okra
- Olives
- Onions
- Purslane Verdolaga
- Squash
- Tomatillo
- Turnip Greens
- Wakame
- Watercress
- Wild Arugula
- Zucchini

Dr. Sebi Fruit List

While the vegetable list is decently lengthy, the fruit list is more restricted, and many types of fruits aren't allowed to be consumed while on the Dr. Sebi diet. However, the fruits list is still offers followers of the diet a diverse set of options. For example, all varieties of berries are allowed on the Dr. Sebi food list except cranberries, which are a manmade fruit. The list also includes:

- Apples
- Bananas
- Berries
- Cantaloupe
- Cherries
- Currants
- Dates
- Figs
- Grapes
- Limes
- Mango
- Melons

- Orange
- Papayas
- Peaches
- Pears
- Plums
- Prickly Pear
- Prunes
- Rasins
- Soft Jelly Coconuts
- Soursoups
- Tamarind

Dr Sebi Food List Spices and Seasonings

- Achiote
- Basil
- Bay Leaf
- Cayenne

- Cloves
- Dill
- Habanero
- Onion Powder
- Oregano
- Powdered Granulated Seaweed
- Pure Sea Salt
- Sage
- Savory
- Sweet Basil
- Tarragon
- Thyme
- Alkaline Grains
- Amaranth
- Fonio
- Kamut

- Quinoa
- Rye
- Spelt
- Tef
- Wild Rice
- Alkaline Sugars and Sweeteners
- Date Sugar from dried dates
- 100% Pure Agave Syrup from cactus

Dr Sebi Herbal Teas

- Burdock
- Chamomile
- Elderberry
- Fennel
- Ginger
- Red Raspberry
- Tila

Dr. Sebi Herb List

The herb list is the most limited of Dr. Sebi's food lists, as it is difficult to find an herb that has not been altered. A good rule of thumb for the herbs is to think of ones that can be used as soon as they are picked from the garden (a non-GMO garden, of course). Some of the most versatile herbs on the Dr. Sebi Herb list include:

- Basil
- Dill
- Oregano
- Onion powder
- Pure sea salt
- Cayenne

Why You Need to Cut Back On Processed and Animal-Based Products

You've probably heard time and time again that processed food is bad for you. "Avoid preservatives; avoid processed foods"; however, no one ever really gives you any real or solid information on why you should avoid them and why they are dangerous. So let's break it down so that you can fully understand why you should avoid these culprits. They have huge addictive properties As humans, we really have a strong tendency to be addicted to certain foods, but the fact is that it's not entirely our fault. Practically all of the unhealthy eats we indulge in, from time to time, activate our brains dopamine neurotransmitter. This makes the brain feel "good" but only for a short period of time. This also creates an addiction tendency; that is why someone will always find themselves going back for another candy bar – even though they don't really need it. You can avoid all this by removing that stimulus altogether.

They are loaded sugar and high fructose corn syrup

Processed and animal-based products are loaded with sugars and high fructose corn syrup which have close to zero nutritional value. More and more studies are now proving what a lot of people suspected all along; that genetically modified foods cause gut inflammation which in turn makes it harder for the body to absorb essential nutrients. The downside of your body failing to properly absorb essential nutrients, from muscle loss and brain fog to fat gain, cannot be stressed enough.

They are loaded with refined carbohydrates

Processed foods and animal-based products are loaded with refined carbs. Yes, it is a fact that your body needs carbs to provide energy to run body functions. However, refining carbs eliminates the essential nutrients; in the way that refining whole grains eliminates the whole grain component. What you are left with after refining is what's referred to as "empty" carbs. These can have a negative impact on your metabolism by spiking your blood sugar and insulin levels.

They are loaded with artificial ingredients

When your body is consuming artificial ingredients, it treats them as a foreign object. They essentially become an invader. Your body isn't used to recognizing things like sucralose or these artificial sweeteners. So, your body does what it does best. It triggers an immune response which lowers your resistance making you vulnerable to diseases. The focus and energy spent by your body in protecting your immune system could otherwise be diverted elsewhere.

They contain components that cause a hyper reward sense in your body

What this means is that they contain components like monosodium glutamate (MSG), components of high fructose corn syrup and certain dyes that can actually carve addictive properties. They stimulate your body to get a reward out of it. MSG, for instance, is in a lot of pre-packaged pastries. What this does is that it stimulates your taste buds to enjoy the taste. It becomes psychological just by the way your brain communicates with your taste buds. This reward-based system makes your body want more and more of it putting

you at a serious risk of caloric overconsumption. What about animal protein? Often times the term "low quality" is thrown around to refer to plant proteins since they tend to have lower amounts of essential amino acids compared to animal protein. What most people do not realize is that more essential amino acids can be quite damaging to your health. So, let's quickly explain how.

Animal Protein Lacks Fiber

In their quest to load up on more animal protein most people end up displacing the plant protein that they already had. This is bad because unlike plant protein, animal protein often lacks in fiber, antioxidants, and phytonutrients. Fiber deficiency is quite common across different communities and societies in the world. In the USA, for instance, according to the Institute of Medicine, the average adult consumes just about 15 grams of fiber per day against the recommended 38 grams. Lack of adequate dietary fiber intake is associated with an increased risk of colon and breast cancers, as well as Crohn's disease, heart disease, and constipation.

What You Stand to Gain from Dr Sebi Diet

The Benefits of Going Plant-Based More and more people are becoming aware of the ability of a whole food plant based diet to help alleviate and even cure many chronic diseases such as heart disease, type 2 diabetes, arthritis, cancers, autoimmune disease, kidney stones, inflammatory bowel diseases and many more. Not to mention, a plant-based diet is more economical – especially when you buy local organic produce that is in season.

Manufactured by Amazon.ca
Bolton, ON